QUICK AND EASY VEGAN RECIPES

Tasty Plant Based Instant Pot Whole Food with Time Saving Meal Plan

Epiphany Hub Prints

TABLE OF CONTENT

INTRODUCTION

Welcome to the savory, compassionate, and straightforward universe! We're about to embark on a culinary excursion that demonstrates that going vegan is not only beneficial to your health and the environment, but it's also incredibly delectable, according to the "Quick and Easy Vegan Recipes" cookbook.

Prepare to unearth a wealth of delectable recipes that will tantalize your palate and transform your kitchen into a plant-powered creative hub. This cookbook is your ticket to simple, delicious, and guilt-free foods that will have you hankering for more, whether you're a seasoned vegan or just starting to explore the world of cruelty-free cuisine.

So get ready to enter into a world where every meal is a celebration of flavor, ethics, and convenience as you roll up your sleeves and sharpen your knives. "Quick and Easy Vegan Recipes" can help you create culinary magic in no time.

THANK YOU VERY MUCH FOR TAKING YOUR TIME TO READ THIS BOOK. I FOUND JOY SHARING MY THOUGHTS WITH YOU. HAVING ENJOYED

"QUICK AND EASY VEGAN RECIPES", I WOULD DROP OUR EMAIL AS A MEANS OF REACHING OUT. MEANWHILE I SENT OUT READING LIST OF MY FAVORITE BOOKS FROM MYSELF AND OTHER AUTHORS ON A WIDE RANGE OF SUBJECTS.

epiphanyhubprints@gmail.com

I ALWAYS HAVE A GIFT FOR EVERYONE THAT REACHED OUT!

CHAPTER ONE

Welcome to the World of Quick and Easy Vegan Cooking

The need for quick, simple, and wholesome meals has never been higher in a world where time seems to fly by more quickly than ever. Finding nourishing food options that promote our health and are consistent with our values and ethics is crucial as we balance our busy lives. Welcome to Quick and Easy Vegan Cooking, a culinary adventure that aims to change the way you perceive plant-based food.

The many possibilities of vegan cuisine are explored in this cookbook, where lively tastes, healthy ingredients, and quick preparation come together to produce meals that are not only delicious but also healthy for the environment and your body.

Whether you're a seasoned vegan trying to expand your recipe collection or someone who is interested in the health advantages of a plant-based diet, these pages are made to motivate and streamline your culinary endeavors.

Advantages of a Vegan Diet

It's important to comprehend why so many people are adopting veganism as a way of life before we get started with the recipes. All animal products, including meat, dairy, eggs, and even honey, are prohibited in a vegan diet. By taking this route, you not only support animal welfare but also gain a variety of health and environmental advantages.

Veganism is praised for its potential to cut cholesterol, decrease the risk of chronic diseases, and support good weight management. Moreover, it considerably lowers your carbon footprint, saving valuable resources and contributing to a planet that is more sustainable. We'll go through these advantages in greater detail so you can see the beneficial effects that your dietary decisions can have on both your health and the environment.

Advice for Easy Vegan Cooking

We recognize that switching to a vegan lifestyle might be intimidating at first, especially if you're used to using conventional ingredients and culinary techniques. We have a section on Tips for Effortless Vegan Cooking as a result. You may get helpful tips on meal planning, ingredient substitutions, and necessary pantry essentials right here. Additionally, we'll share time-saving tips and kitchen tricks to make cooking vegan a breeze.

Therefore, this cookbook has something for everyone, whether you're hoping to adopt healthier, more moral eating habits or are just looking for quick and simple meal options that may accommodate your hectic schedule.

Prepare to set out on a delicious journey into the world of vegan cuisine, where each meal promises to be a beautiful fusion of flavor, practicality, and compassion. Let's investigate the countless possibilities of plant-based food together and learn how it may improve your life, one delectable meal at a time.

PEACE BEGINS ON YOUR PLATE.

-UNKNOWN-

<h1 style="text-align:center">CHAPTER TWO</h1>

In a Flash, Breakfast

We frequently find ourselves looking for a quick and filling breakfast choice in the morning rush. The good news is that going vegan need not mean giving up flavor or nutrition, particularly when it comes to breakfast.

Say goodbye to bland breakfasts and dive into our selection of quick and simple morning treats that will give you a boost of energy and flavor as you start your day.

1.Oats overnighted with a variety of berries

Our Overnight Oats recipe has made mornings much simpler. Rolling oats, your preferred plant-based milk, a little sweetness, and a variety of mixed berries should all be combined in a jar. Before going to bed, place it in the refrigerator so that when you wake up, you'll have a creamy, filling breakfast that is full of fiber, antioxidants, and natural sweetness. It's the ideal grab-and-go choice for those busy mornings.

2.Three variations of avocado toast

With three delicious versions, we're kicking the basic avocado toast up a notch. Your taste buds will dance when you try these concoctions, which range from the traditional avocado and tomato combination to spicy avocado with Sriracha and a sweet variation with avocado and strawberries. To make a breakfast that's not only Instagram-worthy but also a fantastic source of healthy fats and vitamins, all you need is some toasted bread and ripe avocados.

3. Maple-flavored vegan pancakes

The appeal of fluffy, golden pancakes topped with luscious maple syrup is hard to resist. Our vegan pancake recipe ensures a stack of delight that is free of animal products and just as delicious as the classic version. The whole family will enjoy waking up to this breakfast treat, and you'll be amazed at how simple it is to make the ideal pancake.

4. Fruit and Nut Smoothie Bowl

Our Fruit and Nut Smoothie Bowl is a great option if you like to drink your breakfast. Your favorite fruits should be blended with some plant-based yogurt or milk, and some nuts, seeds, and granola should be sprinkled on top for a delightful crunch. It's a personalized nutritional powerhouse that provides vitamins, fiber, and a cool start to your day.

5. Tofu and spinach scramble

Our Tofu Scramble with Spinach is the solution if you are in the mood for a delicious and protein-rich breakfast. In place of eggs, sautéed spinach, crumbled tofu, and a variety of fragrant spices are used in this vegan version of scrambled eggs. You will feel filled till lunchtime with this robust, nourishing option.

You may now enjoy delicious, hassle-free meals that are tailored to your vegan lifestyle and wave goodbye to the morning rush. These dishes are created to be quick, simple, and flavorful, making sure that your day gets off to a good start.

There is something here to suit everyone's tastes, whether they prefer sweet or savory breakfast foods. Get ready for a world of delicious and healthy vegan breakfast options by rising and shining!

YOU CAN'T LOVE ANIMALS AND EAT THEM TOO.

UNKNOWN

CHAPTER THREE

Speedy Soups and Salads

1.Tomato Basil Cream Soup

Enjoy the time-tested solace of a silky tomato soup that has been scented with basil. When you want a warm embrace in a bowl or it's a chilly evening, turn to this quick and simple recipe. A lusciously smooth and dairy-free pleasure is made with fresh tomatoes, fragrant basil, and a tiny bit of coconut milk.

2.Curry soup with chickpeas and vegetables

This healthy chickpea and vegetable curry soup will perk up your day. This soup is the ideal blend of comfort and nutrition because it is full of flavorful ingredients and lively tastes. Chickpeas offer plant-based protein, while a medley of veggies and fragrant spices combines to create a mouthwatering flavor symphony. This soup is just a simmer away from being in a warm bowl.

3.Vegan Caesar salad dressing

With this Caesar salad that is completely vegan-friendly, up your salad game. Using handmade croutons, vegan Caesar dressing, and crisp romaine lettuce, this salad is not only tasty but also guilt-free. Here, the star is the dressing, a savory and tangy creation made entirely of plant-based ingredients that you'll want to spread over everything.

4.Black bean and quinoa salad

This quinoa and black bean salad is the perfect quick and filling meal. It's a nutrient powerhouse that is ready quickly and is packed with protein, fiber, and a rainbow of vegetables. A robust foundation is provided by the fluffy quinoa and filling black beans, and the spicy dressing brings everything together. It is a dish that can be served as a side or a main course.

5.Salad with Mediterranean Couscous

This colorful couscous salad will take your taste senses to the Mediterranean. This salad, which is bursting with tastes and textures, blends light couscous with sun-dried tomatoes, cucumbers, olives, and aromatic herbs. A lemony vinaigrette gives the dish a zingy tang and unifies all the components. Every bite is a lovely taste of the Mediterranean.

These quick and simple vegan dishes demonstrate how straightforward it may be to make flavorful, plant-based meals in addition to being really delicious.

These recipes offer a variety of flavors and textures that will satiate your taste buds and keep you going back for more, whether you're a seasoned vegan or you're just beginning to explore plant-based options. Enjoy these dishes' convenience and sweetness on any occasion!

VEGANISM IS NOT A DIET. IT'S A CHOICE TO SHOW COMPASSION FOR ANIMALS, ANIMALS, THE ENVIRONMENT, AND YOUR HEALTH.

UNKNOWN

CHAPTER FOUR

Lightning-Fast Lunches

1.Vegan BLT Sandwich:

Enjoy the traditional BLT sandwich with a heartfelt twist. Crisp lettuce, juicy tomatoes, smoky tofu or tempeh pieces, and creamy vegan mayo will be used in place of the bacon. For a filling and flavorful sandwich that is cruelty-free and brimming with flavor, layer it all between two cuts of your favorite vegan bread.

2.Noodles with Thai Peanuts:

This quick and simple recipe for Thai peanut noodle will transport your taste buds to Southeast Asia. Tofu or tempeh for extra protein, along with vibrant bell peppers, snappy carrots, and delicate rice noodles, should all be combined. Add crushed peanuts and fresh herbs as a garnish for mouthwatering taste and texture in every bite.

3.Quesadilla with sweet potatoes and black beans:

With these delectable quesadillas, discover a blend of flavors. A delicious filling is made up of roasted sweet potato chunks, spiced black beans, sautéed onions, and vegan cheese. You may prepare the whole thing in a tortilla and heat it until it is crispy and golden, creating a filling lunch or dinner.

4. Hummus with Vegan Wrap:

With this straightforward yet tasty vegan wrap, up your wrap game. Fill a tortilla to the brim with your choice of protein, such as chickpeas or marinated tofu, along with fresh, crunchy vegetables like cucumber, bell peppers, and spinach. For a quick and wholesome on-the-go supper, roll everything up.

5. Jackfruit Sandwich with BBQ:

Prepare to enjoy barbeque flavor without the meat. In this sandwich, the BBQ jackfruit, which has a shredded texture and a smoky-sweet flavor, is the star ingredient. Put it on a bun, top it with some crunchy coleslaw, and sprinkle it with vegan barbeque sauce for a tangy, delicious, and oh-so-satisfying sandwich.

These vegan dishes demonstrate that eating a plant-based diet can be delectable and practical by offering a variety of flavors and textures. With your vegan lifestyle in mind, these meals can accommodate your needs for a light lunch, a big dinner, or a fulfilling snack. Enjoy your culinary adventure!

THE TIME WILL COME WHEN MEN
SUCH AS I WILL LOOK UPON THE
MURDER OF ANIMALS

LEONARDO DA VINCI

CHAPTER FIVE

Effortless Entrées

1.One-Pot Vegan Chili

Warm, hearty, and brimming with flavor, this one-pot vegan chili is a perfect go-to for a quick and satisfying meal. Packed with protein-rich beans, vibrant vegetables, and a blend of aromatic spices, it's a comforting dish that's simple to prepare. Just toss all the ingredients into a single pot, simmer to perfection, and you'll have a steaming bowl of chili ready to enjoy.

2.Lemon Garlic Pasta with Asparagus

In this zesty and vibrant dish, tender asparagus spears meet the bright flavors of lemon and garlic. This lemon garlic pasta with asparagus is a refreshing and quick meal that's perfect for busy weeknights. The combination of fresh, crisp asparagus and tangy lemon zest creates a delightful symphony of tastes, making it a go-to option when you're craving something light and satisfying.

3.Teriyaki Tofu Stir-Fry

For an umami-packed, stir-fried sensation, look no further than this teriyaki tofu stir-fry. It's a fast and flavorful dish that combines crisp vegetables and marinated tofu in a luscious homemade teriyaki sauce. The tofu absorbs the savory-sweet flavors beautifully, and with a quick stir-fry, you'll have a mouthwatering, protein-rich meal that's sure to satisfy your cravings.

4.Vegan Stuffed Bell Peppers

Stuffed bell peppers are a timeless classic, and this vegan version is no exception. Filled with a delectable mixture of grains, legumes, and vegetables, these vegan stuffed bell peppers are a nutritious and delightful option. The peppers roast to perfection, creating a smoky, slightly charred exterior that complements the savory filling. They make an impressive yet easy dish for both everyday dinners and special occasions.

5.Mushroom and Spinach Vegan Lasagna

Indulge in the rich and comforting flavors of lasagna with this mushroom and spinach vegan version. Layers of tender lasagna noodles alternate with a savory mushroom and spinach mixture, all bathed in a creamy vegan béchamel sauce. Baked to golden perfection, this lasagna boasts a satisfying combination of earthy mushrooms, vibrant spinach, and creamy goodness, making it a standout dish in the world of vegan comfort food.

These recipes offer a glimpse into the world of quick and easy vegan cooking, where flavor, nutrition, and convenience come together to create mouthwatering dishes that everyone can enjoy. Whether you're new to vegan cuisine or a seasoned pro, these recipes are sure to become staples in your culinary repertoire.

THE GREATNESS OF A NATION
AND IT'S MORAL PROGRESS CAN
BE JUDGED BY THE WAY ITS
ANIMALS ARE TREATED.

-MAHATMA GANDHI-

CHAPTER SIX

Quick Sides and Snacks

1.Baked Sweet Potato Fries

Crispy, flavorful, and guilt-free, Baked Sweet Potato Fries are a delightful vegan snack or side dish. Sweet potatoes are a nutritional powerhouse, packed with vitamins and fiber.

Here's how to create this tasty treat:

Ingredients:

Sweet potatoes

Olive oil

Salt, pepper, and your choice of seasonings

Preparation:

Preheat your oven.

Cut sweet potatoes into fries or wedges.

Toss them in a mix of olive oil, salt, pepper, and your favorite seasonings.

Spread them evenly on a baking sheet.

Baking:

Bake until they're crispy and golden brown, flipping them once for even cooking.

Serving:

Serve your Baked Sweet Potato Fries with a vegan dipping sauce like garlic aioli or vegan ranch dressing.

2.Crispy Buffalo Cauliflower Bites

Craving the spicy kick of Buffalo wings without the meat? Try Crispy Buffalo Cauliflower Bites. They're a perfect appetizer or snack for parties and game days:

Ingredients:

Cauliflower florets

Flour (use a gluten-free variety if desired)

Plant-based milk

Buffalo sauce

Bread crumbs (or panko for extra crispiness)

Salt and pepper

Preparation:

Dip cauliflower florets into a batter made from flour and plant-based milk, seasoned with salt and pepper.

Roll them in bread crumbs.

Baking:

Bake the coated cauliflower in the oven until they become crispy and brown.

Serving:

Toss the baked cauliflower bites in Buffalo sauce, and serve with vegan ranch or celery sticks.

3.Guacamole and Salsa

Guacamole and Salsa are a classic combo that's quick and easy to prepare. They're perfect for dipping tortilla chips or as a topping for tacos and burritos:

Ingredients:

Ripe avocados

Onion, tomato, cilantro, and lime juice

Salt and pepper

Salsa Ingredients:

Tomatoes, onions, jalapeños, cilantro, and lime juice

Salt and pepper

Preparation:

Dice and mix the ingredients for both guacamole and salsa separately.

Serving:

Serve them with tortilla chips or as condiments for your favorite Mexican dishes.

4.Vegan Spinach and Artichoke Dip

Creamy and savory, Vegan Spinach and Artichoke Dip is a crowd-pleaser at any gathering. Here's how to whip it up:

Ingredients:

Spinach, artichoke hearts, and vegan cream cheese

Garlic, nutritional yeast, and vegan mozzarella

Salt and pepper

Preparation:

Sauté spinach and artichoke hearts with garlic.

Combine them with vegan cream cheese, nutritional yeast, vegan mozzarella, and seasonings.

Baking:

Bake until the dip is bubbly and slightly browned on top.

Serve with tortilla chips, crackers, or fresh vegetable sticks.

5.Roasted Garlic Hummus

Creamy, garlicky, and nutritious, Roasted Garlic Hummus is a versatile dip or spread that's simple to make:

Ingredients:

Chickpeas, tahini, lemon juice, and roasted garlic

Olive oil, cumin, salt, and paprika

Preparation:

In a food processor, combine all ingredients and pulse until well-combined.

Serving:

Serve with pita bread, carrot sticks, cucumber slices, or as a sandwich spread.

CHAPTER SEVEN

Desserts in Minutes

1.Vegan Avocado Chocolate Mousse

Enjoy a creamy, guilt-free chocolate pleasure that is also good for you. It tastes delicious and is a wonderful way to fuel your health while sating your sweet desire with this vegan chocolate avocado mousse.

The deep chocolate taste is delivered by cocoa powder, while avocado gives the thick, silky texture. This dessert, which is naturally sweetened with maple syrup or dates, is a hit with guests and a terrific way to sneak in some healthy components.

2.Peanut butter energy bites without baking

Do you require an instant energy boost? The ideal snack to fuel you throughout the day is these No-Bake Peanut Butter Energy Bites. They give you prolonged energy without the need for baking because they are stuffed with protein, fiber, and healthy fats.

These easy-to-make snacks are made from rolled oats, peanut butter, honey or maple syrup, and optional ingredients like chocolate chips or dried fruit. Create a batch and keep them in the refrigerator for a quick snack that will satiate your hunger.

3.Frozen Yogurt with Mixed Berries

On a hot day, do you want for a cool, refreshing dessert? Look no further than this frozen yogurt with mixed berries. This colorful, delicious treat is so easy to make that you won't believe it.

A creamy, luscious treat made with frozen berries, dairy-free yogurt, and a hint of sweetness is ideal for summer or any time you want a fruity boost. You may indulge guilt-free because it's a healthier alternative to classic ice cream.

4.Rice Krispie Treats for vegans

Do you still have any leftover Rice Krispie Treats from your childhood? Here's a vegan adaptation of that well-liked dish, though! Without using any animal ingredients, these gooey, marshmallow-y, and incredibly delectable vegan Rice Krispie Treats are made.

You can quickly reproduce this childhood favorite using plant-based butter substitute and vegan marshmallows. They are ideal for gatherings, school lunches, or just to satiate your sweet tooth.

5.Simple chocolate chip cookies that are vegan

Without the traditional Easy Vegan Chocolate Chip Cookies, no collection of vegan desserts would be complete. Your go-to recipe for scrumptious, chewy, chocolatey cookies that are also vegan will be this one.

You may enjoy these cookies with a glass of almond milk or a cup of tea because they use dairy-free chocolate chips and straightforward plant-based replacements. They'll be a hit with vegans and non-vegans equally, so bake a batch and share the love.

These vegan dishes will satisfy your cravings for a guilt-free delight, an energizing snack, a cool treat, a childhood favorite, or a traditional dessert. They demonstrate that you may take advantage of classic recipes' flavor without sacrificing your vegan lifestyle or your ethical principles. Prepare to prepare these delectable treats and satiate your palate the vegan way!

TO BECOME VEGETARIAN IS TO
STEP INTO THE STREAM WHICH
LEADS TO NIRVANA.

-BUDDHA-

CHAPTER EIGHT

Weeknight Dinner Solutions

Tips for Meal Preparation and Batch Cooking

For sustaining a healthy and sustainable vegan lifestyle, meal planning and batch cooking are essential techniques. They let you to always have a great and nourishing dinner available while saving time and decreasing food waste. To keep you on track, consider the following advice on meal planning and batch cooking:

Plan Your Weekly Menu: Consider spending some time each week planning your menu. Build your menu around the ingredients you currently have in your cupboard and refrigerator. As a result, less food will be wasted.

Create a Shopping List: After you've thought through your food plan, make a shopping list. To avoid impulsive purchases and to make sure you have all the components on hand, follow it as strictly as you can.

Ingredient Preparation: Spend some time beforehand chopping, washing, and preparing the ingredients. Making quick meals over the week will be lot simpler if you already have the vegetables, grains, and proteins prepared.

Batch Cook Staples: Cooking staples in bulk involves cooking bigger quantities of grains (such as rice, quinoa, and pasta), beans, and legumes. These can be used as the foundation for a variety of recipes and can be frozen or refrigerated in parts.

Use Freezer-Friendly Containers: Spend money on freezer-safe containers of high quality. Your batch-cooked meals or ingredients should be portioned out into these containers, which should be marked with the date. You can keep track of what is in your freezer using this.

Ideas for Vegan Meal Prep

Your life can be made simpler by prepping vegan meals, especially during hectic workweeks. Here are some suggestions for vegan meal preparation:

Mason jar salads: To assemble a salad in a mason jar, layer the dressing at the bottom and then layers of grains, vegetables, and greens. Just shake it when you're ready to eat, then indulge.

Overnight Oats: Prepare overnight oats in pots using your preferred plant-based milk, oats, and garnishes like fruits, nuts, and seeds. In the morning, they'll be prepared for quick grab-and-go.

Vegan Stir-Fry Kits: Chop up a variety of vegetables and tofu, then place them in different containers for vegan stir-fry kits. Serve them over rice or noodles after stir-frying them in your preferred sauce.

Smoothie Packs: Put your smoothie ingredients in freezer bags in advance. Simply empty the bag into your blender, add liquid, and start blending when you're ready.

Vegetarian soups and stews can be made in large quantities, portioned out, and frozen for convenient lunches or meals.

Weeknight Dinner Menus that Are Simple and Quick

Having a few go-to supper menus can come in handy on weeknights when you're busy. Following are some quick and simple vegan supper dish suggestions:

Menu 1:

Teriyaki Tofu Stir-Fry for the entrée

Steamed broccoli as a side

Vegan chocolate avocado mousse for dessert

Menu 2:

Vegan Chickpea Curry for the starter.

Basmati Rice on the side

Dessert: Frozen Yogurt with Mixed Berries

Menu 3:

Vegan BBQ as an entrée Sandwich with Jackfruit

Baked sweet potato fries as a side

No-Bake Peanut Butter Energy Bites for dessert

These menus feature foods that cook quickly and need little preparation, making them ideal for hectic evenings. You are welcome to mix and match foods to suit your preferences for flavor and diet. Have fun cooking!

CONCLUSION

Our adventure through "Quick and Easy Vegan Recipes" has been nothing short of wonderful in the rich realm of plant-based cooking. From colorful salads to filling main dishes and decadent desserts, we've figured out how to make amazing vegan treats that are both quick and healthy.

Remember that every meal you cook puts you one step closer to living a better, more environmentally friendly, and compassionate lifestyle as you enjoy the last pages of this cookbook. These dishes offer countless options, and your culinary explorations are only getting started.

So let's keep the stovetops sizzling, the ovens baking, and those aprons on. You are not only sustaining your body but also the earth and a better future with each delicious creation. We appreciate your participation in this delicious adventure. May your kitchen always be a place of inspiration, happiness, and delectable vegan magic.

HAVE FUN COOKING!